PILATES
FOR SENIORS

Expert Gentle Exercises For Flexibility, Strength, And Pain Relief – Enhance Mobility, Improve Balance, And Boost Overall Health With Tailored Workouts For Older Adults

ROBERT LUGO

CHAPTER 1 4

Introduction To Pilates For Seniors 4

CHAPTER 2 10

Getting Started With Pilates 10

CHAPTER 3 14

Pilates Fundamentals For Seniors 14

CHAPTER 4 17

Essential Pilates Exercises For Seniors 17

CHAPTER 5 23

Progressing In Pilates Practice 23

CHAPTER 6 26

Special Considerations For Seniors 26

CHAPTER 7 30

Mindfulness And Relaxation In Pilates 30

CHAPTER 8 34

Nutrition And Wellness For Seniors 34

CHAPTER 9 38

Pilates For Long-Term Health And Independence 38

CHAPTER 10 42

Community And Support 42

CHAPTER 11 45

Faqs And Common Concerns 45

CHAPTER 12 49

Case Studies And Success Stories 49

Conclusion 52

CHAPTER 1
Introduction To Pilates For Seniors

Pilates for seniors represents a holisctic approach to fitness and well-being that is specifically tailored to meet the unique needs and capabilities of older adults. This form of exercise focuses on enhancing core strength, flexibility, balance, and overall body awareness through controlled movements and mindful breathing techniques. Unlike more high-impact exercises, Pilates offers a gentle yet effective way for seniors to improve their physical health while also promoting mental clarity and relaxation.

Recognising the Fundamentals of Pilates:

Central to the practice of Pilates is its core principles, which guide the execution of exercises and contribute to its effectiveness for seniors. These guidelines consist of flow, breath, precision, centering, focus, and control.

Concentration involves focusing the mind on each movement to ensure proper execution and maximize benefits. Control emphasizes the importance of performing exercises with smooth, deliberate movements to avoid strain or injury. Centering focuses on engaging the core muscles, particularly the abdominal and pelvic floor muscles, to support posture and stability. Precision involves performing each movement with accuracy and attention to detail, which enhances effectiveness and reduces the risk of overexertion.

Breath plays a vital role in Pilates, with practitioners instructed to coordinate movements with deep, diaphragmatic breathing to enhance relaxation, oxygenation, and mindfulness. Finally, flow refers to the seamless transition between exercises, creating a continuous and fluid movement sequence that promotes endurance and grace. Understanding and applying these principles is essential for seniors to derive maximum benefit from their Pilates practice, fostering a sense of physical well-being, mental focus, and overall vitality.

Benefits of Pilates for Seniors:

The benefits of Pilates for seniors are multifaceted, addressing both physical and mental aspects of health and well-being. One of the primary advantages is improved core strength, which is crucial for maintaining stability, balance, and posture as individual's age.

By strengthening the deep abdominal muscles and the muscles supporting the spine, Pilates helps seniors prevent falls, reduce back pain, and enhance overall mobility and functionality in daily activities.

Flexibility is another key benefit of Pilates, as the exercises promote the elongation of muscles, joints, and connective tissues, leading to an increased range of motion and ease of movement. This is particularly beneficial for seniors who may experience stiffness or joint discomfort, as Pilates can help alleviate these issues and improve overall flexibility and mobility.

In addition to physical benefits, Pilates offers significant mental and emotional advantages for seniors. The mindful approach to movement and breath awareness promotes relaxation, stress reduction, and a sense of mental clarity and focus.

This can be especially beneficial for seniors dealing with anxiety, depression, or cognitive decline, as Pilates provides a positive outlet for improving mood, enhancing cognitive function, and promoting overall well-being.

Safety Considerations and Modifications:

When introducing Pilates to seniors, safety considerations and modifications are paramount to ensure a positive and effective experience. Seniors may have specific health concerns, mobility limitations, or physical challenges that require adjustments to the exercises. Instructors and practitioners alike need to prioritize safety and make appropriate modifications as needed.

One key aspect of safety in Pilates for seniors is proper alignment and posture. Emphasizing correct alignment helps prevent strain on joints and muscles, reduces the risk of injury, and maximizes the benefits of each exercise. This includes maintaining a neutral spine, engaging the core muscles, and avoiding excessive strain or overextension.

Another important consideration is the pace and intensity of the exercises. Seniors may need a slower pace and gentler approach to allow for proper technique and avoid fatigue or overexertion. Gradually progressing in difficulty and intensity as seniors build strength and confidence is crucial for a safe and sustainable Pilates practice.

Additionally, instructors should be mindful of any pre-existing conditions or injuries that seniors may have and tailor exercises accordingly. This may involve using props or modifications to accommodate individual needs, such as using a chair for support, adjusting the range of motion, or providing alternative exercises that target the same muscle groups without exacerbating existing issues.

By prioritizing safety, making appropriate modifications, and encouraging open communication between instructors and seniors, Pilates can be a safe, enjoyable, and highly beneficial form of exercise for older adults, promoting physical fitness, mental well-being, and overall quality of life.

CHAPTER 2
Getting Started With Pilates

Assessing Readiness for Pilates Practice

Before seniors embark on a Pilates journey, it's crucial to assess their readiness for this form of exercise. Unlike high-impact workouts, Pilates is gentle on the joints and focuses on controlled movements, making it suitable for many seniors. However, individual health considerations must be taken into account. Seniors should consult their healthcare provider before starting any new exercise regimen, including Pilates, especially if they have pre-existing medical conditions or mobility issues.

Assessing readiness involves evaluating factors such as overall health, physical fitness level, flexibility, and any existing injuries or limitations. Seniors should be aware of their body's capabilities and limitations to ensure a safe and effective Pilates practice.

A thorough assessment can help determine the appropriate starting point and tailor Pilates exercises to meet individual needs.

Setting Up a Safe and Comfortable Practice Space

Creating a conducive environment is essential for seniors to enjoy and benefit from Pilates practice. The practice space should be well-lit, ventilated, and free from obstacles to minimize the risk of accidents or injuries. Seniors should choose a quiet and peaceful area where they can focus and concentrate on their movements without distractions.

A non-slip mat or padded surface is recommended to provide comfort and support during Pilates exercises. The mat should be firm enough to support the body but not too hard to cause discomfort. Additionally, having props such as resistance bands, Pilates balls, and foam rollers can enhance the Pilates experience and add variety to workouts.

Choosing Appropriate Clothing and Equipment

Seniors should wear comfortable and breathable clothing that allows for ease of movement during Pilates sessions. Loose-fitting but not overly baggy clothes are ideal to ensure freedom of movement without getting tangled or hindered by excess fabric. It's important to choose moisture-wicking fabrics to keep the body dry and comfortable, especially during longer workout sessions.

When it comes to Pilates equipment, seniors can start with the basics such as a Pilates mat, resistance bands, and small props like Pilates balls or foam rollers. These tools can enhance the effectiveness of exercises and provide added resistance or support as needed. Seniors should also consider investing in supportive footwear, especially if they have foot or ankle issues, to ensure stability and safety during Pilates movements.

By assessing readiness, setting up a safe practice space, and choosing appropriate clothing and equipment, seniors can embark on their Pilates journey with confidence and enjoy the many benefits this form of exercise has to offer.

CHAPTER 3
Pilates Fundamentals For Seniors

Pilates, renowned for its focus on core strength, flexibility, and overall body conditioning, holds particular relevance for seniors. This age group often seeks exercises that are gentle yet effective in promoting mobility, balance, and a sense of well-being. Pilates, with its emphasis on controlled movements, breathwork, and mind-body connection, aligns well with the needs and goals of seniors.

Breathing Techniques in Pilates

One of the foundational aspects of Pilates is its emphasis on mindful breathing. For seniors, mastering proper breathing techniques can significantly enhance the benefits of Pilates exercises. Deep diaphragmatic breathing, often referred to as "Pilates breathing," involves inhaling through the nose, expanding the ribcage and abdomen, and exhaling fully to engage the core muscles.

This controlled breathing not only oxygenates the body but also promotes relaxation, reduces stress, and enhances focus during Pilates sessions.

Core Engagement and Stability

For seniors, maintaining a strong and stable core is essential for functional movement and injury prevention. Pilates excels in targeting the core muscles, including the abdominals, back extensors, and pelvic floor muscles.

Through a series of exercises that emphasize core engagement, such as the Pilates Hundred, leg circles, and pelvic tilts, seniors can improve their posture, balance, and overall stability.

Strengthening the core also supports spinal alignment, which can alleviate discomfort and improve mobility, particularly beneficial for seniors dealing with age-related changes in their musculoskeletal system.

Proper Alignment and Posture

As seniors often face challenges related to posture and alignment due to factors like sedentary lifestyles or age-related changes, Pilates offers a systematic approach to improving body awareness and alignment. Exercises focusing on spinal articulation, such as the Pilates roll-up and spine stretch forward, encourage seniors to lengthen their spine, engage their core, and maintain proper alignment throughout movements.

This emphasis on alignment not only enhances the effectiveness of Pilates exercises but also translates into improved posture in daily activities, reducing the risk of strains or injuries.

In conclusion, Pilates fundamentals for seniors encompass mindful breathing techniques, core engagement and stability, and proper alignment and posture. These foundational elements not only enhance the physical benefits of Pilates but also contribute to overall well-being, mobility, and quality of life for seniors engaging in this practice.

CHAPTER 4
Essential Pilates Exercises For Seniors

Gentle Warm-Up Exercises:

When delving into Pilates exercises for seniors, a crucial starting point is gentle warm-up exercises. These exercises serve as a preparatory phase, priming the body for more intense movements while reducing the risk of injury. In a senior-friendly Pilates routine, warm-up exercises focus on improving circulation, enhancing joint mobility, and awakening muscle groups gradually. Examples of gentle warm-up exercises include:

1. Neck Rolls: Slowly rotate the head in a circular motion, first clockwise and then counterclockwise, to loosen neck muscles and improve range of motion.

2. Shoulder Circles: Lift the shoulders towards the ears, then roll them back and down in a circular motion, promoting flexibility and relieving tension in the shoulders and upper back.

3. Arm Swings: Extend arms to the sides and swing them gently back and forth, engaging the shoulder joints and promoting blood flow to the arms.

4. Hip Circles: Stand with feet hip-width apart and rotate the hips in circular motions, loosening hip joints and improving mobility in the lower back and hips.

5. Ankle Circles: Sit or stand and lift one foot off the ground, then rotate the ankle in clockwise and counterclockwise circles to improve ankle flexibility and circulation.

These gentle warm-up exercises set the foundation for a safe and effective Pilates session, allowing seniors to ease into more challenging movements with increased comfort and reduced risk of strain.

Mat Exercises for Strength and Flexibility:

Mat exercises are fundamental in Pilates for seniors, focusing on building strength, improving flexibility, and enhancing overall body control. These exercises can be modified to suit varying fitness levels and mobility challenges, making them accessible and beneficial for seniors. Key mat exercises for seniors include:

1. Pelvic Tilts: Lie on the back with knees bent and feet flat on the mat. Gently tilt the pelvis backward and forward, engaging the core muscles and promoting lumbar spine flexibility.

2. Leg Circles: While lying on the back, lift one leg toward the ceiling and make circular motions with the foot, enhancing hip mobility and strengthening the lower abdominals.

3. Bridge Pose: Begin lying on the back with knees bent and feet hip-width apart. Lift the hips off the mat, creating a bridge shape with the body, to strengthen the glutes, hamstrings, and lower back.

4. Spine Twist: Sit on the mat with your legs extended. Twist the upper body to one side while reaching the opposite arm behind, promoting spinal mobility and stretching the obliques.

5. Swan Dive: Lie facedown on the mat with arms extended overhead. Lift the upper body and legs simultaneously, engaging the back muscles and improving spinal extension.

These mat exercises target core strength, balance, and flexibility, essential components for seniors looking to maintain mobility and functional independence.

Chair-Based Pilates Exercises for Mobility:

For seniors with limited mobility or those who prefer seated exercises, chair-based Pilates offers a valuable approach to improving flexibility, strength, and overall mobility. These exercises can be performed using a sturdy chair with a backrest for support. Chair-based Pilates exercises for seniors include:

1. Seated Marches: Sit upright in a chair and lift one knee toward the chest, then alternate with the other knee, mimicking a marching motion. This exercise improves lower body circulation and strengthens the hip flexors.

2. Seated Side Stretch: Sit with feet flat on the floor and arms extended overhead. Lean gently to one side, stretching the obliques, then return to the center and repeat on the other side.

3. Chair Leg Extensions: Sit at the edge of the chair with the back straight. Extend one leg forward, then lower it back down, alternating between legs to strengthen the quadriceps and improve leg mobility.

4. Chair Yoga Twists: Sit tall in the chair and twist the upper body to one side, using the chair's backrest for support. Hold the twist briefly, then return to the center and repeat on the other side to enhance spinal mobility.

5. Seated Chest Opener: Sit with hands clasped behind the back and gently lift the chest upward, opening the shoulders and stretching the chest muscles.

Chair-based Pilates exercises offer a seated alternative that promotes flexibility, strengthens muscles, and enhances overall mobility, making them ideal for seniors seeking safe and effective workout options.

Incorporating these essential Pilates exercises for seniors into a regular fitness routine can yield significant benefits, including improved posture, enhanced balance, increased muscle tone, and a greater sense of overall well-being. By focusing on gentle warm-up exercises, mat exercises for strength and flexibility, and chair-based Pilates exercises for mobility, seniors can experience the transformative power of Pilates in promoting healthy aging and active lifestyles.

CHAPTER 5
Progressing In Pilates Practice

Progressing in Pilates practice for seniors involves several key concepts that contribute to an effective and fulfilling workout experience.

By advancing exercises for increased challenge, incorporating props for variety, and utilizing methods to track progress and set goals, seniors can optimize their Pilates practice for improved strength, flexibility, and overall well-being.

Advancing exercises for increased challenge is crucial in maintaining progression and preventing plateaus in Pilates practice. Seniors can achieve this by modifying traditional exercises to add complexity or intensity. For example, starting with basic movements like pelvic tilts and gradually progressing to more advanced variations such as leg circles or single-leg stretches challenges both stability and strength. Incorporating equipment like resistance bands or Pilates rings can also add resistance and engage different muscle groups, providing a more dynamic workout experience.

Another essential aspect of progressing in Pilates practice for seniors is the strategic use of props for variety. Props such as stability balls, foam rollers, and small Pilates balls can enhance exercises by adding instability or targeting specific muscle groups. For instance, using a stability ball during exercises like bridges or squats requires seniors to engage their core muscles for balance, thereby enhancing core strength and stability. Additionally, props like foam rollers can be utilized for myofascial release, improving flexibility and reducing muscle tension.

Tracking progress and setting goals are integral parts of any fitness regimen, including

Pilates for seniors. Seniors can track their progress by keeping a workout journal or using fitness tracking apps to record their exercises, repetitions, and any modifications made.

This helps in monitoring improvements over time and identifying areas for further development. Setting realistic and achievable goals, such as increasing the number of repetitions or holding a plank for a longer duration, provides seniors with motivation and a sense of accomplishment in their Pilates journey.

Overall, progressing in Pilates practice for seniors involves a thoughtful approach that combines challenging exercises, varied props, and effective progress tracking. By incorporating these concepts into their routine, seniors can experience enhanced strength, flexibility, and overall fitness, leading to a healthier and more active lifestyle.

CHAPTER 6
Special Considerations For Seniors

Special Considerations for Seniors in Pilates involve a nuanced understanding of the aging process and its impact on physical health. This section delves into key aspects such as addressing common concerns like joint stiffness and balance issues, modifying exercises for specific conditions such as arthritis and osteoporosis, and emphasizing the importance of regular practice and consistency.

One of the primary concerns for seniors engaging in Pilates is joint stiffness. As people age, joint mobility can decrease due to factors like reduced synovial fluid production and changes in cartilage composition. Pilates offers a gentle yet effective approach to improve joint flexibility. Exercises focusing on controlled movements, stretching, and fluid motions can help lubricate joints, reduce stiffness, and enhance overall mobility.

Emphasizing proper alignment and technique is crucial to prevent strain on joints and maximize the benefits of Pilates for seniors.

Balance issues are another common consideration for seniors, especially as the risk of falls increases with age. Pilates exercises that promote core strength, proprioception, and stability can significantly improve balance and reduce the likelihood of falls. Incorporating exercises that challenge balance, such as standing on one leg or performing movements on unstable surfaces like a balance pad, can enhance proprioceptive awareness and improve overall balance control. Moreover, Pilates encourages mindful movement and body awareness, which are essential for seniors to maintain stability and prevent falls in daily activities.

Modifying exercises for specific conditions is paramount in Pilates for seniors. Conditions like arthritis and osteoporosis require tailored approaches to ensure safety and effectiveness. For individuals with arthritis, low-impact exercises that focus on gentle movements and joint mobility are recommended. Modifications such as using props like cushions or resistance bands to support joints can alleviate discomfort while still allowing seniors to benefit from Pilates. Similarly, seniors with osteoporosis benefit from exercises that promote bone density and strength without risking fractures.

Pilate's exercises emphasizing spinal alignment, weight-bearing movements, and controlled resistance can help maintain bone health and reduce the risk of osteoporotic fractures.

Consistency and regular practice are fundamental principles for seniors engaging in Pilates. Unlike sporadic workouts, consistent Pilates practice yields long-term benefits, including improved strength, flexibility, balance, and posture. Encouraging seniors to establish a regular Pilates routine, ideally incorporating sessions several times a week, enhances muscle memory, motor skills, and overall fitness levels. Consistency also fosters a sense of discipline and commitment, which are essential for sustaining a healthy and active lifestyle in later years.

Special considerations for seniors in Pilates encompass addressing joint stiffness and balance issues, modifying exercises for specific conditions like arthritis and osteoporosis, and emphasizing the importance of regular practice and consistency. By tailoring Pilates workouts to suit the needs and capabilities of seniors, instructors, and practitioners can promote optimal physical health, mobility, and well-being in the aging population.

CHAPTER 7
Mindfulness And Relaxation In Pilates

In Pilates for seniors, the integration of mindfulness techniques is a pivotal aspect that transcends mere physical exercise, delving into the realms of mental and emotional well-being. Mindfulness, rooted in ancient practices like yoga and meditation, has found a contemporary home in Pilates studios worldwide. This fusion of mindful awareness with the precise movements of Pilates creates a transformative experience, offering seniors not just physical fitness but also mental clarity and emotional balance.

The incorporation of mindfulness techniques into Pilates practice involves a conscious and focused approach to each movement. It starts with the breath—the rhythmic inhalations and exhalations that synchronize with the flow of exercises. Seniors are encouraged to deepen their awareness of the breath, using it as a guide to connect the mind with the body. This mindful breathing serves as a constant anchor, grounding individuals in the present moment and fostering a sense of calmness amidst the physical exertion.

As seniors engage in Pilates movements with mindfulness, they begin to cultivate a heightened sense of body awareness. This heightened awareness goes beyond simple physical alignment; it involves a deep understanding of how each movement affects the body, from the subtle shifts in posture to the engagement of specific muscles. Through mindful movement, seniors learn to move with intention and precision, avoiding unnecessary strain or tension.

One of the key benefits of incorporating mindfulness into Pilates for seniors is the profound relaxation and stress reduction it offers. Mindful movement promotes relaxation by encouraging seniors to let go of tension held in the body. As they focus on the present moment and the sensations within their bodies, they naturally release physical and mental stress. This relaxation response not only enhances the overall Pilates experience but also contributes to better sleep quality, reduced anxiety, and improved mood.

The mind-body connection in Pilates takes on a deeper significance when coupled with mindfulness practices. Seniors learn to move with awareness, bringing conscious attention to each part of their bodies engaged in the exercises.

This mind-body connection fosters a sense of unity, where movements are not just mechanical but meaningful expressions of self-awareness and self-care. Through mindful Pilates practice, seniors develop a profound understanding of their bodies' capabilities and limitations, empowering them to move with grace and ease.

In conclusion, mindfulness and relaxation are integral components of Pilates for seniors, enriching their physical, mental, and emotional well-being. By incorporating mindfulness techniques into Pilates practice, seniors can experience a holistic approach to fitness that nurtures not just their bodies but also their minds and spirits. This fusion of mindful awareness with the precise movements of Pilates creates a transformative experience, offering seniors not just physical fitness but also mental clarity and emotional balance.

CHAPTER 8
Nutrition And Wellness For Seniors

Nutrition plays a vital role in the overall well-being of seniors, influencing their health, energy levels, and quality of life. As individuals age, their nutritional needs may change, making it crucial to pay attention to dietary habits and choices. Understanding the importance of nutrition for seniors involves considering factors such as hydration, balanced diet composition, and the role of complementary wellness practices like meditation and sleep hygiene.

One of the primary reasons why nutrition is essential for seniors is its impact on maintaining physical health and functionality. Adequate nutrition provides the body with essential nutrients, vitamins, and minerals necessary for proper organ function, tissue repair, and immune system support. For seniors, whose bodies may experience age-related changes like reduced muscle mass, weaker bones, or slower metabolism, a well-rounded diet becomes even more critical.

Hydration is a fundamental aspect of nutrition that is often overlooked but holds significant importance for seniors. Dehydration can lead to various health issues, including urinary tract infections, kidney stones, and even cognitive impairment. Therefore, encouraging seniors to consume an adequate amount of water throughout the day is essential. Additionally, incorporating hydrating foods such as fruits, vegetables, and soups into their diet can contribute to overall hydration levels.

Diet tips tailored specifically for seniors can help them make healthier choices and meet their nutritional needs. These tips may include recommendations such as consuming a variety of colorful fruits and vegetables to ensure a diverse nutrient intake, incorporating lean proteins like fish, poultry, beans, and nuts for muscle health, and opting for whole grains over refined carbohydrates for sustained energy levels.

Portion control and mindful eating practices are also valuable for maintaining a healthy weight and digestive wellness.

In addition to focusing on dietary aspects, seniors can benefit from complementary wellness practices that promote overall well-being. Meditation, for instance, has been shown to reduce stress, improve mental clarity, and enhance emotional resilience. Encouraging seniors to engage in mindfulness exercises or relaxation techniques can have positive effects on their mental and emotional health, contributing to a sense of calm and inner balance.

Sleep hygiene is another crucial component of wellness for seniors. Quality sleep is essential for cognitive function, mood regulation, and physical recovery. Educating seniors about the importance of a consistent sleep schedule, creating a relaxing bedtime routine, and optimizing their sleep environment (e.g., comfortable mattress, dark and quiet room) can help improve sleep quality and overall wellness.

Nutrition and wellness are interconnected aspects of senior health that require attention and proactive management. By emphasizing the importance of balanced nutrition, adequate hydration, and incorporating complementary wellness practices like meditation and sleep hygiene, seniors can enhance their overall well-being, maintain vitality, and enjoy a higher quality of life as they age.

CHAPTER 9
Pilates For Long-Term Health And Independence

Pilates stands out as a holistic approach to enhancing long-term health and fostering independence among seniors. Its core principles of breath, concentration, control, centering, precision, and flow contribute significantly to overall well-being. As individuals age, maintaining physical fitness becomes paramount for sustaining an active lifestyle and preserving independence. Pilates, with its focus on strengthening core muscles, improving flexibility, and enhancing balance, emerges as an invaluable tool in this journey toward long-term health and independence.

Creating a Sustainable Pilates Routine

The cornerstone of reaping lasting benefits from Pilates lies in creating a sustainable routine tailored to individual needs and capabilities.

Seniors embarking on a Pilates journey should start by consulting with qualified instructors who understand the unique requirements of older adults. Establishing a routine that integrates Pilates sessions into weekly schedules ensures consistency, allowing seniors to experience gradual improvements in strength, flexibility, and overall well-being. Incorporating a variety of Pilates exercises, including mat-based and equipment-based workouts, adds diversity and prevents monotony, keeping seniors engaged and motivated in their fitness journey.

Setting Long-Term Fitness Goals

Setting realistic and achievable long-term fitness goals is essential for seniors engaging in Pilates. Goals should be specific, measurable, attainable, relevant, and time-bound (SMART), catering to individual fitness levels and aspirations.

For example, a senior may set a goal to improve core strength, increase flexibility, or enhance balance over a designated period.

Working closely with Pilates instructors, seniors can develop personalized fitness plans that align with their long-term goals, ensuring steady progress and continuous motivation. Regular progress assessments and adjustments to goals further optimize the Pilates experience, empowering seniors to track their achievements and stay committed to their fitness journey.

Celebrating Milestones and Achievements

Celebrating milestones and achievements is a vital aspect of sustaining motivation and fostering a positive outlook on fitness. Seniors engaged in Pilates should acknowledge and celebrate every milestone, whether it's mastering a challenging exercise, improving flexibility, or achieving better posture. Recognizing progress, no matter how small reinforces a sense of accomplishment and encourages seniors to stay dedicated to their Pilates practice. Instructors play a crucial role in providing positive reinforcement, offering encouragement, and highlighting the significance of each achievement, fostering a supportive and empowering environment for seniors on their fitness journey.

Pilates offers seniors a pathway to long-term health and independence through sustainable routines, well-defined fitness goals, and the celebration of milestones and achievements. By embracing Pilates as a holistic approach to fitness, seniors can enhance their physical well-being, improve their quality of life, and maintain independence well into their golden years.

CHAPTER 10
Community And Support

Group Pilates classes for seniors offer a multitude of benefits that extend beyond physical fitness. These classes provide a supportive environment where individuals can come together to improve their health and well-being. One of the key advantages of participating in group Pilates sessions is the sense of community and support that it fosters among seniors.

Firstly, let's delve into the specific benefits of participating in group Pilates classes for seniors. These classes are designed to cater to the unique needs and capabilities of older adults, focusing on gentle yet effective exercises that promote strength, flexibility, and balance. Unlike individual workouts, group classes offer a social setting where seniors can interact with like-minded individuals, fostering a sense of camaraderie and motivation.

Building a supportive fitness community is crucial for seniors embarking on a Pilates journey. In a group setting, participants often develop friendships and bonds with classmates, creating a supportive network that extends beyond the studio. This sense of belonging and connection can have a profound impact on mental well-being, reducing feelings of isolation and loneliness commonly experienced by older adults.

Moreover, the social aspects of Pilates for seniors go beyond the physical workout. These classes provide an opportunity for social interaction, conversation, and shared experiences, contributing to overall happiness and life satisfaction. Group Pilates sessions often incorporate partner exercises or group activities, further enhancing the social dynamics and creating a fun and engaging atmosphere.

In addition to the physical and social benefits, group Pilates classes for seniors offer a sense of accountability and encouragement. Being part of a group motivates individuals to stay consistent with their workouts and pushes them to challenge themselves in a supportive environment. The encouragement and positive reinforcement from instructors and peers can boost confidence and self-esteem, empowering seniors to achieve their fitness goals.

Overall, the community and support aspect of group Pilates classes play a pivotal role in enhancing the overall well-being of seniors.

These classes not only improve physical fitness but also foster social connections, emotional support, and a sense of belonging, making them a valuable component of a holistic approach to senior health and wellness.

CHAPTER 11
Faqs And Common Concerns

Answering common questions about Pilates for seniors involves delving into various aspects that often arise as seniors consider incorporating Pilates into their fitness routines. One of the primary questions is about the safety of Pilates for seniors, especially those with pre-existing conditions or limited mobility. Pilates, when done correctly and under proper guidance, can be safe and beneficial for seniors. However, it's essential to consult with a healthcare professional before starting any new exercise program, including Pilates, to ensure it aligns with individual health needs and goals.

Another common query revolves around the effectiveness of Pilates for seniors in improving flexibility and strength. Pilates emphasizes core strength, flexibility, and balance, which are crucial for seniors to maintain independence and reduce the risk of falls.

It can help improve posture, joint mobility, and overall body awareness, making it a valuable addition to a senior's fitness regimen. Moreover, Pilates can be adapted to suit varying fitness levels and physical abilities, making it accessible and beneficial for seniors of all backgrounds.

Addressing myths and misconceptions about Pilates for seniors is vital in promoting its understanding and acceptance among this demographic. One prevalent myth is that Pilates is only for the young or those already fit and flexible. In reality, Pilates is a low-impact exercise that can be modified to accommodate seniors with different fitness levels and mobility challenges. It focuses on controlled movements, proper alignment, and breath awareness, making it suitable for seniors looking to improve their overall fitness and well-being.

Another misconception is that Pilates requires expensive equipment or extensive studio sessions. While Pilates equipment such as reformers and resistance bands can enhance workouts, many Pilates exercises can be done using only a mat or basic props, making it accessible for home practice. Additionally, Pilates classes for seniors are often available at community centers, senior centers, or online platforms, providing affordable options for those interested in this form of exercise.

Troubleshooting tips for beginners in Pilates for seniors can help address common challenges and ensure a positive and enjoyable experience.

One common issue is discomfort or pain during certain movements, which may indicate incorrect form or excessive strain. Seniors should focus on proper alignment, start with gentle movements, and listen to their bodies to avoid overexertion. Gradually increasing intensity and difficulty levels can also help seniors progress safely in their Pilates practice.

Another common challenge is consistency and motivation, especially for seniors who may be new to regular exercise or facing health-related barriers. Setting realistic goals, tracking progress, and finding enjoyable Pilates routines can boost motivation and adherence. Seniors can also benefit from group classes or virtual communities where they can connect with peers, share experiences, and stay motivated together.

Addressing FAQs and common concerns about Pilates for seniors involves providing accurate information, dispelling myths, and offering practical tips for a safe and enjoyable experience. Pilates can be a valuable exercise option for seniors seeking to improve flexibility, strength, balance, and overall well-being, and with proper guidance and adjustments, it can be tailored to meet the diverse needs of seniors at different fitness levels.

CHAPTER 12
Case Studies And Success Stories

Case studies and success stories play a vital role in understanding the impact of Pilates on seniors' health and well-being. These narratives provide tangible evidence of how Pilates can positively influence the lives of older adults, addressing various physical, mental, and emotional aspects. Through real-life examples, inspirational stories, and testimonials, the transformative power of Pilates for seniors becomes evident.

Real-life examples of seniors benefiting from Pilates showcase the diverse range of improvements experienced by individuals engaging in this practice. These examples may include seniors who have struggled with mobility issues, chronic pain, or age-related conditions such as osteoporosis or arthritis. By incorporating Pilates into their routine, these individuals have reported enhanced flexibility, increased strength, and improved posture.

For instance, a case study might focus on an elderly individual who, after consistent Pilates sessions, noticed a significant reduction in joint pain and an ability to perform daily activities with greater ease.

Inspirational stories highlight the emotional and psychological benefits of Pilates for seniors. Beyond the physical improvements, many older adults find renewed confidence, a sense of accomplishment, and a positive outlook on life through their Pilates practice.

These stories may feature seniors who initially felt discouraged or limited by their age but discovered newfound resilience and vitality through Pilates. For example, a senior participant might share how Pilates not only improved their physical health but also boosted their self-esteem and motivation to stay active.

Testimonials from participants offer firsthand accounts of the impact of Pilates on seniors' overall well-being. These testimonials often reflect on specific aspects such as increased energy levels, better sleep quality, reduced stress, and enhanced mental clarity. Seniors may express gratitude for discovering Pilates as a holistic approach to maintaining their health and vitality as they age. For instance, a testimonial might highlight how Pilates helped a senior individual regain balance and coordination, leading to a more independent and fulfilling lifestyle.

These case studies, success stories, and testimonials collectively contribute to a comprehensive understanding of Pilates as a beneficial practice for seniors.

They showcase the multifaceted advantages of Pilates, from physical rehabilitation and pain management to emotional resilience and improved quality of life.

By sharing these real-life experiences, the narrative of Pilates for seniors expands beyond theoretical concepts, illustrating its tangible and profound effects on individuals' lives.

Conclusion

Pilates for seniors is not just about exercise; it's a journey towards holistic wellness and independence. By embracing the core principles of Pilates, seniors can unlock a myriad of benefits, from improved strength and flexibility to enhanced mental focus and relaxation.

Getting started with Pilates is about more than just physical readiness. It's about creating a safe and inviting space where seniors can comfortably engage in their practice, wearing the right clothing and using appropriate equipment to support their movements.

The fundamentals of Pilates for seniors lie in mastering breathing techniques, engaging the core for stability, and maintaining proper alignment and posture throughout exercises. These foundational aspects ensure that seniors can derive maximum benefit while minimizing the risk of injury.

From gentle warm-up exercises to mat routines focusing on strength and flexibility, and chair-based exercises for mobility, the journey through essential Pilates exercises is tailored to the unique needs of seniors, allowing for gradual progression and adaptation as abilities improve.

As seniors progress in their Pilates practice, they can explore advanced exercises, incorporate props for variety, and set goals to track their progress over time. Consistency and regular practice are emphasized, laying the foundation for long-term health and independence.

Special considerations, such as addressing joint stiffness and balance issues or modifying exercises for specific conditions like arthritis or osteoporosis, ensure that Pilates remains accessible and beneficial for seniors of all abilities.

The integration of mindfulness and relaxation techniques adds a dimension of mental well-being to Pilates practice, promoting stress reduction, improved focus, and a deeper mind-body connection in movement.

Nutrition and wellness are essential components of the Pilates journey for seniors, with emphasis placed on proper hydration, diet tips, and complementary practices like meditation and sleep hygiene for overall well-being.

Looking towards the future, Pilates for seniors is not just about the exercises—it's about creating a sustainable routine, setting long-term fitness goals, and celebrating every milestone and achievement along the way.

Community and support play a vital role in the Pilates experience, with group classes offering camaraderie, motivation, and a supportive environment where seniors can thrive together, enjoying the social aspects of fitness alongside physical benefits.

Answering common questions, dispelling myths, and providing troubleshooting tips ensure that seniors feel confident and empowered in their Pilates journey, knowing that they have the knowledge and resources to overcome any challenges.

Finally, real-life case studies and success stories serve as inspirational reminders of the transformative power of Pilates for seniors, showcasing the tangible improvements in health, mobility, and overall well-being that are achievable through dedication and commitment to this practice.

www.ingramcontent.com/pod-product-compliance
Lightning Source LLC
Chambersburg PA
CBHW050243230526
45470CB00005B/2093